THE 20TH-CENTURY PLAGUE

The numbers already dying from AIDS worldwide are worrying enough. But many more are infected with the virus. In the 1990s the situation will be far worse. But how much worse? Just how bad is AIDS going to be?

Dr Collier uses the most up-to-date figures to show how rapidly this epidemic can spread. She highlights the ominous social and economic results if the worst happens, with not enough young adults to care for the elderly and to parent a full next generation.

With the help of other experts, she points to the only real solution. And her book describes just how this can be found. She also shows how a person can enjoy a safe lifestyle.

Some of her conclusions contradict present policies. So the substance of this book has been sent as an open letter to leaders of opinion in government, the media, schools.

Dr Collier has had seven years in general practice. Early in 1985 she became deeply concerned about AIDS, and she is now AIDS Lecturer and Resource Officer for the Christian Medical Fellowship, which is an association of Christian doctors whose aims include pursuing the highest standards in Christian and professional life.

Copyright © 1987 Christian Medical Fellowship

Published by
Lion Publishing plc
Icknield Way, Tring, Herts, England
ISBN 0 7459 1453 5
Albatross Books Pty Ltd
PO Box 320, Sutherland, NSW 2232, Australia
ISBN 0 86760 962 1

First edition 1987

British Library Cataloguing in Publication Data

Collier, Caroline
 The twentieth century plague
 1. AIDS (Disease)
 I. Title
 616.9′792   RC607.A26

 ISBN 0 7459 1453 5

Printed and bound in Great Britain
by Cox and Wyman Ltd, Reading

THE 20th CENTURY PLAGUE

DR CAROLINE COLLIER

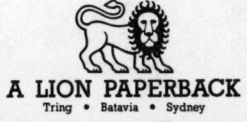

A LION PAPERBACK

Tring • Batavia • Sydney

The author is indebted for the material in chapter 7 to the Revd David Field, Vice Principal of Oak Hill Theological College, London, and for parts of chapter 6 to Dr John Guillebaud, MA, FRCS, FRCOG, Medical Director of the Pyke Centre, Westminster, and Senior Lecturer/Consultant, Department of Gynaecology, UCM School of Medicine, and Dr H.E. Larson, MD, FRCP, of the Medical Research Council Scientific Staff.

Contents

Charts and statistical tables

1

A Deafening Silence

Flying through the dawn skies of astonishing beauty over the Arabian Sea, it was good to have left behind the grey skies of England and the bitter cold of February, 1985. From the snowdrifts in Shropshire I was travelling into the sunshine of an Australian summer. We descended through 10,000 feet of dense cloud and landed in Sydney. There we met a wall of heat, streams of healthily tanned bodies in the streets, the screeching of sulphur-crested cockatoos and galahs—and news of the AIDS epidemic.

I had my first introduction to AIDS as I read the newspaper headlines at breakfast: morning after morning they focused on AIDS. I noticed a pile of books on a news-stand in the centre of the city, and saw they were books about AIDS. But I was not ready to buy one yet. I decided to wait until I got home to England.

For some days I travelled with an Australian friend who was making a kind of farewell tour, saying goodbye to people before leaving on an assignment overseas. Our trip took in a town 200 miles inland from Sydney. I learnt that a previous church youth club leader, who had left for England some years before, had recently died of AIDS as chaplain to Chelmsford Prison. The people of the town had loved this man, yet I was struck by the fear and bewilderment on their faces as his name was mentioned. That was my second introduction to the AIDS epidemic.

Later I was able to visit a doctor working in community medicine. I asked him what was happening with the AIDS epidemic.

'All I know is that the numbers are doubling every six months,' he told me. I felt chilled as I received my third introduction to AIDS.

Back in England I looked for books on the epidemic and found none. I waited for newspaper articles and television programmes on AIDS, but there were none. Soon I discovered that for every person with AIDS it was estimated that between fifty and a hundred more were infected. I read in the medical journals the occasionally published figures for AIDS, and set them alongside what I had heard in Australia of the six-month doubling time. It was clear that we were heading for an epidemic of major proportions. And it seemed that no one, in Britain at least, was taking it seriously.

A year passed. I met a retired television producer and we talked for a while about AIDS. I told him that the most important thing was to interest the television networks in the epidemic, for them to have the facts then available. I became involved in writing down what I knew about AIDS and, more importantly, what we should be doing about it. This report was circulated round the television networks and I heard no more. But now I was moving on from my passive interest in AIDS. It was time for me actively to come to grips, in my work and my thinking, with the massive threat posed by this disease.

In November 1986 I was asked to write a general information paper on AIDS, and started to look at the wider implications of the epidemic for the future, both nationally and internationally. This book has grown from there.

2

Plague

Epidemic diseases have been known to humanity for many thousands of years. Some have been localized, affecting a small geographical area, while others have been widespread, affecting large parts of the world. Epidemics on a large scale do not happen with great frequency, and so they have often caught both doctors and governments unprepared.

It will be helpful to put AIDS in the context of previous large-scale epidemics. When we see how governments and people in general have reacted in the past, it may give some clues to likely reactions to this twentieth-century plague.

Endemic diseases

Epidemic diseases are those which suddenly appear, sweep across an area of population, and then disappear. But most illnesses, the ones from which a large part of humanity is condemned to suffer, are not like that. These are the endemic diseases, which remain entrenched within a population.

There are six main endemic diseases for which the World Health Organization has special projects:

• **Leprosy** is one. It is thought that there are 15

million people suffering from this disease, only 5 million of whom receive treatment.

- **Malaria** causes sickness and death on a large scale. Tens of millions are infected with it.
- **Schistosomiasis** (bilharzia) affects vast numbers: some 180 to 200 million people.
- **Chagas disease**, a form of sleeping sickness caused by the trypanosome parasite, makes 7 million people ill.
- **Filariasis**, caused by a parasitic worm, is bad news in India where 150 million people are at risk, as are 30 million in China.
- **Onchocerciasis** is found mainly in Central and West Africa. 250,000 people are blind because of this disease while up to 20 million are infected.

All these diseases are avoidable and curable and, where resources are available, they cease to be a problem. AIDS is different from these. It is an epidemic disease; there is no evidence of it being self-limiting; there is no immunity to it; and there is no means of cure. The World Health Organization has described the AIDS pandemic as 'a health problem of extraordinary scope and unprecedented urgency . . . that has been seriously underestimated and underappreciated.'

Epidemic diseases

The Plague of Justinian began in Arabia, reaching Egypt by AD 542. It caused great damage to the Eastern Roman Empire of Justinian and crossed to Europe during the following decades. It finally reached England in the year 664, over 120 years after its appearance in Arabia. Four or five generations of people in Britain would have regarded the plague—if they had known of its existence—as far removed from their experience, not a threat to them.

The Black Death is perhaps the best-known world epidemic. It began in 1346 and spread through India, Tartary, Mesopotamia, Syria and Armenia. By 1347 it had reached Hungary, Italy and Spain; a year later France and Germany. It finally arrived in England in 1349. It had run its course in three years, but by then it had killed one third of Europe's inhabitants. The Black Death was followed by sporadic outbreaks of bubonic plague throughout the next three centuries, one of these being the Great Plague of 1665 in London.

Epidemics of meningitis occurred in France and Germany in 1482. There were outbreaks of the 'Sweating Sickness', causing considerable mortality, in 1485, 1499, 1506, 1517 and 1551.

Syphilis first appeared in Europe in an epidemic form at the end of the fifteenth century. The most learned physicians of that period described it as a new disease which they had never seen before. The disease spread rapidly through Italy, and appeared in France, Germany and Switzerland in 1495. It had reached Holland and Greece by 1496, and a year later England and Scotland. It finally arrived in Hungary and Russia in 1499.

The syphilis plague is an important one to look at as in some respects it prefigures the AIDS epidemic. It was a new disease, spread mainly through sexual means. It was also thought to be spread by the public bath-houses and after syphilis appeared many of these were closed. It spread widely in some countries for more than four years before other countries saw any cases at all. The terrible tragedy of congenital infection was found to occur, a mother infected with syphilis passing it to her baby in the womb. People became so conscious of syphilis that many other conditions were confused with it and wrongly attributed to it. People who were infected with syphilis and infectious to others passed it on while they still seemed healthy, before the severe crusting, disfiguring sores appeared which identified them as syphilitic.

Syphilis was untreatable; there was then no cure. Ultimately it was usually fatal, sometimes after years of illness. It spread widely in the population of Europe.

The most recent pandemic broke out in 1918 in a world already decimated by war. In twelve weeks one billion people, half the world's population at the time, were affected by virulent influenza. Twenty-two million died.

Cholera epidemics have now become past history in Europe, while smallpox, once the scourge of whole areas, has now been eradicated. In the nineteenth century 400,000 Europeans were dying from smallpox every year, and by the mid-twentieth century between 10 and 15 million people in thirty-three countries were infected, with 2 million people dying from it every year. After a campaign lasting ten years the World Health Organization finally tracked down the last case of smallpox and eradicated the disease in 1975.

What common factors can we see in people's reactions to these fearful epidemics?

Denial and fear

People's first response to an impending disaster of great magnitude is often to deny it. This has been so with epidemic diseases in the past and many would maintain that the common reaction during the early years of the AIDS epidemic has been one of denial. The reasons for this are threefold:

● **The human brain does not want to accept that something terrible is happening**.
● **The authorities want to prevent panic**, and so they may at first refuse to acknowledge the situation publicly.
● **To admit that a disaster is coming means taking action to avert it**. If for any reason that action cannot be decided upon or cannot be implemented, then denial is the easiest official course.

In the seventeenth century, in *A Treatise of the Plague*, Thomas Lodge wrote:

'If by chance, or by the will of God, the city becometh infected, it ought not incontinently to be made known; but those that have the care and charge of such as are attainted ought in the beginning to keep it close, and wisely conceal the same from the common sort.'

Secrecy or denial embodies in itself the desperate hope that perhaps, after all, the thing feared will go away.

Fear is another common response to disaster threatening. Historically this has shown itself in flight, running away from infected areas to safer, non-infected parts. Fear has also been demonstrated in violence and debauched behaviour.

Persecutions and massacres were common across Europe during the fourteenth century, around the time of the Black Death. And in more recent years, during the outbreak of Kuru in New Guinea in which large numbers of women and children of the Fore tribe died, sorcery was blamed and revenge, hate and murder caused the deaths of many people.

The desire for action

When once the temptation to deny a danger is overcome, there follows a desire to do something to avert it. This action may sometimes be quite inappropriate. During the bubonic plagues of the Middle Ages, groups of people were made scapegoats. People also thought it would help to carry sweetsmelling pomanders.

But sometimes the action is appropriate to the danger.

Surveillance was first undertaken by the great Greek doctor, Hippocrates. He wrote the First and Third Books of Epidemics and, together with his son, left four volumes of notes on epidemic diseases. But his studies were not followed up in the centuries following his death in 377 BC.

Public Health Measures against plague were first developed in Europe during the fourteenth century. Plague arrived in Venice in January 1348, and two months later the Venetians appointed a special cabinet committee of three noblemen to consider what measures should be taken. These special measures included:

- New burial places away from the city
- A special service of barges to carry the dead
- The dead to be buried at least five feet underground
- The release of all debtors from gaol
- Strict control of immigration and shipping
- Quarantine stations, where the sick and those surviving the disease were isolated for forty days. Quarantine also included travellers and goods from infected areas.

In 1399 there was fumigation during plague, houses were ventilated and the bedding of those who had died from plague was burned. People were not allowed to live in plague houses for a period of time following the death of the victims.

During the following few decades many cities throughout Europe followed the lead set by these early public health measures. Yet it was to be over 300 years before Bills of Health were generally instituted in the year 1665.

Today, in facing the AIDS pandemic which may prove even more serious than almost any previous plague, we need to learn from history.

The first lesson is not to deny the reality of the danger. The months of silence of which I became aware in 1985 were a bad start. When people are properly informed, they will begin to co-operate in preventive measures.

The next is that such measures need to cover whole societies. Epidemics are no respecters of boundaries.

But yet each plague is unique, AIDS not least of all. In some ways it is like no illness we have seen before. There is no way to protect ourselves from it apart from avoiding infection. Its only limiting factor lies in the number of people exposed to it. And there is no known cure.

3

A New Disease

In 1986 the Chief Medical Officer of Britain's Department of Health and Social Security, Sir Donald Acheson, issued a warning:

> Controlling the spread of infection must be regarded as an issue of prime importance to the future of the nation.

Again, Otis Bowen, United States Secretary of Health, has said,

> AIDS could well become one of the worst health problems in the history of the world . . . an awesome health problem that could involve millions of people who are going to die as a result.

And Director General Dr Halfdan Mahler, of the World Health Organization, puts it like this:

> We stand nakedly in front of a pandemic as mortal as any pandemic there has ever been.

So plainly AIDS is going to be serious, more serious than the layperson can easily visualize in what are still the early days of this epidemic's spread.

AIDS is a new disease which was first recognized in 1981 and has been reported in 127 countries. The World Health Organization estimates that by 1991 there will be between 50 and 100 million people worldwide infected with the Human Immunodeficiency Virus, HIV. This is a conservative estimate, in that it assumes Asia and Latin America will not be badly affected. It is now thought that the majority of these 50 to 100 million will develop AIDS. The numbers infected will continue to rise, doubling every six to twelve months. So by the late 1990s the situation may be much worse even than this WHO estimate suggests.

In September 1986 *The Times* of London carried a grim warning:

From the speed with which the Acquired Immune Deficiency Syndrome (AIDS) virus is spreading through Africa, America and Europe it is clear that mankind is on the threshold of a viral catastrophe. Unless doctors and scientists reappraise their approach, its impact on man within twenty years cannot fail to match that of the Black Death in the fourteenth century, and the world wars of this century.

The aim of this book is to begin to sketch out the lines of just such a reappraisal. Just how should people and governments be dealing with this impending catastrophe? I am going to examine various options, and finish with definite proposals. In particular, I have set out to show the national and economic implications of 'best' and 'worst' scenarios.

And also, as a Christian doctor funded by the Christian Medical Fellowship, I point out that there are important roles that Christians and churches can play.

But before moving on to any of that, we need to stop for a moment and see clearly what is the special character of this new disease which makes it so uniquely dangerous.

What is AIDS?

AIDS is the result of a virus, the Human Immunodeficiency Virus, or HIV for short. When this virus infects a person it destroys the body's natural defence mechanism against other infections. The virus attacks one of the cells in the body which maintain these defences. After entering the cell the virus multiplies and causes inactivation or destruction of these cells, and as they are destroyed a person eventually becomes unable to recover from infections. At this point the person is said to have the Acquired Immune Deficiency Syndrome, AIDS.

The virus can attack other cells as well. For example, it attacks the brain cells causing brain damage of varying degree from forgetfulness or change of character to dementia. Many patients dying of AIDS have signs of brain damage.

Where is AIDS found?

The new disease of AIDS has now been reported in 127 countries since 1981. North and South America, Western and Eastern Europe, Africa, Australia and South and East Asia all have people who have been infected with the virus (see the chart on page 21).

AIDS in the West

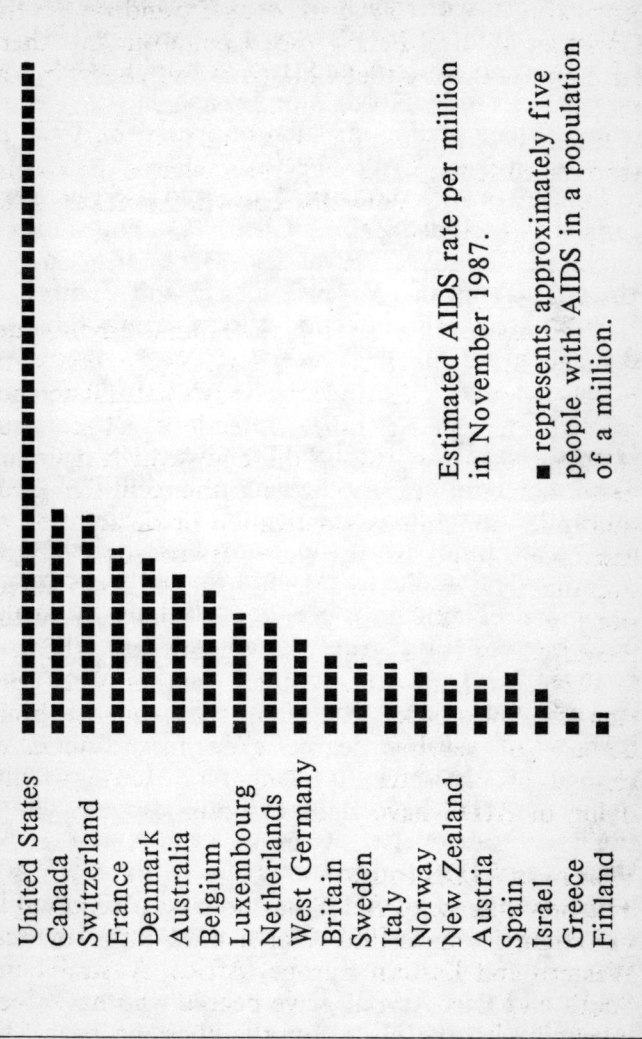

Estimated AIDS rate per million in November 1987.

■ represents approximately five people with AIDS in a population of a million.

United States
Canada
Switzerland
France
Denmark
Australia
Belgium
Luxembourg
Netherlands
West Germany
Britain
Sweden
Italy
Norway
New Zealand
Austria
Spain
Israel
Greece
Finland

The speed with which AIDS is spreading varies in different countries. The spread is rapid in tropical Africa, South America and the Caribbean, while it is slower in Europe, North America and Japan. We are going to look at this question of spread in detail in chapter five.

The African countries where AIDS is very common include Zaire, Chad, Congo, Central African Republic, Rwanda, Burundi, Gabon, Uganda, Tanzania, Malawi, Kenya and Zambia.

In all areas HIV infection affects mainly those in the age group 18–49 years, the years of greatest sexual activity.

How does HIV infection spread?

The virus is found in semen, vaginal fluids, blood, saliva, breast milk, cerebrospinal fluid, bone marrow, joint fluid, tears and transplanted tissues. It may also be found in faeces and urine if these contain any blood. The main routes of spread are by sexual intercourse or by sharing contaminated needles and syringes. Only semen, vaginal fluids, blood and transplanted tissues have conclusively been shown to transmit the virus.

Contaminated blood products caused some people to become infected with the virus and this was a most tragic early development. Many haemophiliacs and some recipients of blood transfusions were infected before testing of blood started in the United States in March 1985, and in Britain in October of the same year.

More recently, in 1987, three health-care workers in the United States have been shown to have been infected with HIV after exposure of their skin to the blood of infected patients. This discovery has important implications for all health work. (Two of these workers were only picked up because they were routinely tested as blood donors.)

Once infected with this virus a person remains infected for the rest of his or her life. People who are infected with HIV are also infectious to others. They are able to transmit the virus to others by means of sexual intercourse or by their blood. Women may transmit the virus to their babies during pregnancy or childbirth, or occasionally by breastfeeding.

In non-African countries the virus has spread fastest among homosexuals and intravenous drug abusers. However, in Africa, where there is very little homosexuality, the virus has spread widely in the heterosexual population. Heterosexual spread is also occurring in Europe and the United States, although the heterosexual epidemic seems to be at a relatively early stage in Western countries. This leads to one of the most difficult questions in predicting how fast AIDS is going to spread. How soon and how widely will the African type of heterosexual spread be repeated in the West?

Can AIDS be cured?

Unlike other viruses, HIV is able to hide itself inside cells for long periods, sometimes many years, before causing disease. The virus is also able to change the composition of its surface easily, making it difficult to produce a vaccine.

The antibodies which an infected person produces in response to HIV do not have the ability to destroy the virus. So the antibodies are helpful in testing for the disease, because they serve to identify an infected individual whose blood when tested shows antibody-positive. But a person cannot get rid of the infection in the same way that other infections are overcome.

HIV attacks a specialized group of white blood cells called T-helper or T4 cells. The virus kills or immobilizes these cells which are then unable to perform that part of their job which involves recognizing foreign substances (antigens) and initiating defensive action to deal with them.

It now appears that there are T4 receptors on some brain cells. The virus crosses into the brain and may directly attack brain cells. This is thought to be the cause of the dementia which is now recognized as a complication of HIV. Some patients become increasingly confused, showing symptoms akin to senility.

HIV was at first thought to be a fragile virus. But now it is known to be quite persistent. It can survive in an infectious form for more than seven days in a dry state, and more than fifteen days in a wet state.

There are four main ways of killing the virus:

- **Autoclaving** (steam sterilizing), at 134°C for three minutes at 2.1 kg/cm^2 (220.8 kPa), or at 121°C for fifteen minutes at 1.05 kg/cm^2 (103 kPa);
- **Boiling**—laundering at 95°C for ten minutes;
- **Using bleach**—at 1 part bleach per 10 parts water (the same as Domestos) when the contamination is heavy, or 1 part bleach per 100 parts water (as Milton Sterilizer) when it is light. The potentially HIV-carrying article should be immersed for thirty minutes.

● **Using glutaraldehyde**, freshly activated two per cent solution, immersing the contaminated material for three hours.

Once the HIV virus has penetrated a cell, it is transcribed into double-stranded DNA, in other words it becomes part of that cell's genetic information. This means it is very difficult to eradicate the virus. This is an extremely hard disease to cure. In fact a medical solution to AIDS would herald a new era in medicine.

This is not easy for laypeople to accept and cope with, perhaps because cures have been found for so many things that we have come to expect a cure for everything. But accept it we must. A cure for AIDS almost certainly lies well in the future. The emphasis now and in the coming years must be on prevention more than cure.

The stages of infection
There are three main stages, which may take years to work through.

● **The symptomless stage** comes first. When a person is initially infected with the virus there are usually no symptoms, and there may be no symptoms for many months or some years. The normal defence system of the body produces some antibodies to HIV. This process takes some weeks and usually causes no symptoms, although a few people will have a glandular-fever-like illness when first infected, or occasionally symptoms affecting the nervous system. Usually the person appears quite healthy during this stage. But of course this presents a major danger because although a person may feel perfectly well, he or she can still infect other people with the virus.

The only certain way of knowing whether a person is infected is through testing the blood for antibodies to HIV. We will look at testing in detail in chapter 8.

● **Signs and symptoms** begin to appear at a second stage, perhaps as much as seven years after infection. Two sets of symptoms are most common.

Persistent generalized lymphaderopathy (or PGL) is a condition in which there are swollen lymph nodes in two or more sites (excluding the groin region) for longer than three months.

AIDS related complex (ARC) includes weight loss, loss of appetite, night sweats, fever, skin rashes, diarrhoea, lack of resistance to infection and tiredness. Most who have ARC will go on to develop AIDS.

● **AIDS itself** is the third stage. For most people infected with HIV the final stage is reached when the body's immune (defence) system is destroyed, allowing rare infections to invade that person and eventually cause death. Common infections may also invade the person with AIDS and cause unpleasant symptoms.

People with AIDS can have a wide variety of symptoms and secondary diseases. Some symptoms are the result of damage to the immune system and some are due to the virus' effect on other parts of the body. These diseases include:

—**Chest infection**, with pneumocystis carinii or tuberculosis;

—**Brain infection**, which may take one of two forms. The brain may be directly attacked by HIV; or there

may be opportunistic infections or brain tumours causing symptoms. There may be encephalitis, meningitis, fits, paralysis, dementia, even blindness.
—**Bacterial or protozoal diseases of the gut**. These may result in diarrhoea caused by various organisms (cytomegalovirus, salmonella, cryptosporidium and isosporidium), difficulty in swallowing because of candida (thrush) in the oesophagus, or ulceration around the anus.
—**Various forms of cancer**. These include Kaposi's sarcoma (purple lumps and blotches), Non-Hodgkins lymphoma, carcinoma of the tongue and anus, or Hodgkins disease.
—**Skin problems**, such as recurrent cold sores, recurrent shingles, ringworm, folliculitis, or boils in the groin and armpits.

This is by no means an exhaustive list. Because the body's defences are suppressed, patients may develop any of a number of bacterial, viral, fungal or protozoal infections. AIDS can be a horrible illness.

AIDS and the brain

HIV may directly attack the brain and nervous system, with or without the presence of opportunistic infections. Symptoms of AIDS encephalopathy (damage to the brain) include forgetfulness, loss of concentration, attention problems, disorientation in time and place, behavioural changes, agitation, a psychotic state, fits and focal neurological signs. Signs of AIDS encephalopathy include paralysis, slowness of speech or of movement, altered moods, difficulty maintaining balance, fits, tremor, difficulty in articulating speech or in swallowing, disinhibited behaviour, or a person becoming stuperozed and confused.

Blindness caused by cytomegalovirus sometimes occurs as the retina is damaged by this virus.

The brain effects of HIV have important implications. The judgment and skills of a person flying a jet, for example, or driving a public vehicle may be impaired. Also miners, lift-shaft operators, HGV drivers and those working in heavy construction may become a danger to others. Of special importance are those in the Armed Forces whose work involves nuclear or conventional weapons and national security. Or the decision-making ability of someone involved with important business negotiations or international relations may be similarly affected. It would affect people deciding about housing and health as well! Of course this problem occurs wherever brain damage develops, but we are going to see it much more frequently with the growth of AIDS.

Seventy-five per cent of people presenting for the first time with AIDS will have a life-threatening illness; half of these will be a chest infection, usually caused by pneumocystis carinii.

Once a person has developed AIDS, he or she will almost certainly be dead within three years.

How far is the disease likely to spread? We return to that crucial question in chapter 5. But before that, we need to look at how people with AIDS can be adequately cared for.

4

People Not Statistics

There is inevitably a lot in this book about figures. This is always so in studies of epidemics. But each unit in each table represents a person, sick and in need of care.

The sick have a very special place within society. Whatever the nature or cause of the disease or disability, the person concerned is surrounded by other people wanting to help, to nurse and to comfort. To care is a human instinct.

To some extent this help has become formalized and institutionalized in many societies today, so that we have come to think in terms of hospitals, hospices, hostels, home-care teams and voluntary workers. However, these are only the visible, public forms of caring. The tremendous amount of care given by families to family members or to neighbours by neighbours is unquantifiable. It is this deep well of selfless love and compassionate care which binds communities together and enriches both those who care and those who are cared for.

People who have had their immune systems damaged by HIV and are particularly vulnerable to diseases will have varying degrees of illness, and a wide variety of symptoms. Some will be physically weak and emaciated, some will be blind, some incontinent, some showing signs of brain damage. All will be having to cope with the knowledge of a shortened life expectancy and an uncertain pattern of illness. Although most people with AIDS will at times experience the more visible, public forms of caring such as hospitals and home-care teams, by far their biggest support will be personal care from their families, friends and neighbours.

People who live in a country which has a National Health Service do not have to rely on being able to raise insurance to cover hospital and other medical care, nor on being in employment in order to qualify for a work-linked health-care scheme. To this extent, therefore, the fear of illness being linked to destitution is removed. Political decisions in a country such as Britain forty years ago, and the immense investment in health-care facilities in many countries over the past decades have laid a solid foundation for the medical care which will be needed in this epidemic.

Yet no government can hope to provide all the care needed in the community, and greater emphasis must be placed on 'community' care.

Care and compassion will be required, both communally and on a personal level. The provision of the basic structure of health care is the responsibility of government, and this applies also to the care of people with AIDS. This requires the political will to do it, and a creative, positive attitude to the challenge which the AIDS epidemic presents. But AIDS also presents a personal challenge to all of us, and this will be met in many different ways.

Some people will care for members of their own

families as they become ill with AIDS: sons and daughters, brothers or sisters, perhaps even parents. They will do whatever needs to be done—washing, providing meals, changing sheets and generally keeping the sufferer comfortable. Friendship, love and companionship as well as gentleness and patience will be a part of that care. In the same way some people will look after neighbours and members of other people's families.

Part of the caring will be towards people who will eventually die. But part will be caring for children whose parents will have died. This will be a different commitment involving the total giving of oneself as parents for a lifetime.

In this new epidemic, because of the age group of those mainly affected and the long period of time before developing the disease for many of those infected, new approaches may be appropriate. For instance, a family with both parents and one or two children affected, and perhaps one or two non-infected children, could be 'bonded' with a childless couple. This couple could be 'aunt and uncle', helping during the varied illnesses which will ensue and finally adopting the remaining child or children after the parents' death. In this way the future adoptive parents will have shared in the care of the original parents, will have come to be trusted by those parents, and will have shared in the bereavement of the children. We are looking here at something far more extensive than simply adoption.

There are many other ways of caring. Some who will not feel able to nurse, clean or cook for someone with AIDS, could do the housework of someone who *is* able to do these things, so freeing that person to do the frontline caring. Others may offer hospitality to the family and loved ones of someone with AIDS, if that person is in hospital far from home.

Preparing for the future

It is possible to begin now to prepare oneself for a caring role in the future. For those interested in developing basic nursing skills, these can be taught in courses locally. The beginnings of networks of care may be set up with small groups getting to know each other, becoming knowledgeable about AIDS and sharing skills and friendship, perhaps for several months before those skills are actually used. The important thing is to be ready when the care is needed.

As the epidemic progresses, some countries may adopt segregation of those who are HIV-positive and those with AIDS. In this situation care and compassion will be no less important. Most of those who are HIV-positive will look and feel healthy. By the time they develop signs of illness they will have developed strong bonds of friendship and companionship within the group. Many will also have family living with them who are HIV-negative and these, together with friends and others, may care for them during periods of illness and in their last days. Under this policy the best possible medical care can be provided as resources can be concentrated in the area in which they are most needed. In a segregated situation, sufferers will not feel the isolation which sometimes comes from that secrecy and anonymity which may in mixed communities prevent the full support of a person with AIDS.

In a society where those infected with HIV are separated from the population at large, there will already have been painful partings, very parallel to the pain of bereavement itself. This pain will have come many months or years earlier than would otherwise have occurred. It will be rather like the separation which happens during time of war as men and sometimes women are called up for active service.

And yet the powerful motivation of protecting the nation will in part lessen the pain, whether the danger is from epidemic or whether it is from war.

Care and compassion will be needed whether or not policies of separation are followed.

What the church can do

The world faces a disaster of unprecedented magnitude in the AIDS epidemic. And, as in all disasters, the church has a vital role to play. It is important that it is united in this—united in the love of Christ in caring for the souls, bodies and minds of people in society today.

The sheer scale of the pandemic will call for human resources of care and compassion beyond what society normally has to provide, and the church is one possible pool from which such resources could be drawn. It already has manpower and experience in several of the relevant areas.

Planning

In a united approach to the AIDS epidemic, Christian churches of all denominations could join together in planning so that Christian resources are seen to be released for people who most need them.

What kind of resources does the church have to offer? Buildings for a start. But also publishing resources, Christian workers and teachers, chaplains in hospitals, and finance which could be used for education and youth projects.

The church has had a long tradition of offering guidance on sexual behaviour and relationships, and this will be very much needed. Christians will also be called on to assume a higher profile in the pastoral and counselling areas of care.

The church should actively plan to influence public opinion as much and as quickly as possible to change the commonly accepted view—at least in a large part of the younger community—that courting and dating include sexual intercourse. Chastity—waiting until marriage to enjoy the delights of a sexual relationship—and fidelity—being faithful to one lifelong partner—are words which should be frequently heard and seen in print by readers many times a day. These are the two kinds of behaviour which will totally protect people from AIDS, and these concepts need to be widely understood.

The church should plan to set a higher priority on youth work, because this is going to be a highly vulnerable generation. Christian youth clubs and youth workers are needed more than ever before. In a situation of high youth unemployment it should be remembered that boredom and poverty can combine to reduce social contacts. Youth clubs can provide enjoyment and an active social life for young people as well as opportunities for personal growth and development in mind, body and spirit. Unemployed youth projects and initiatives can be undertaken as an extension of this youth work.

Christians should plan to pray for the nation and the world in this time of crisis and danger. Prayers about the AIDS epidemic could be regularly included in services, and there could be days of prayer for AIDS. There is much to be prayed for: for altered attitudes and lifestyles, for the success of research being undertaken, for the comfort of people with AIDS and AIDS-related conditions and their loved ones, for the government who is charged with leadership of the nation at this time, and for the church itself that it might grow in wisdom, compassion and love.

The church should plan to reintroduce religious teaching into schools in a more vital way, to prepare teaching aids and materials, and possibly to provide travelling schools speakers on 'sex and religion'.

Perhaps Christians should also plan to encourage a change of emphasis in the media to a less exploitative and more emotionally sensitive attitude to sexuality, promoting the positive value to individuals, to families and to society of lifelong stable relationships.

Warning and teaching
The church has traditionally had a warning role. From ancient times this has been so, and today the danger comes from a disease spread by one of the most vital urges of the human race, the sex drive.

The Christian rules relating to sex, part of the general consensus until twenty or so years ago, do give total safety from the new disease of AIDS. The church therefore has a duty to restate these guidelines today. Christians should be speaking clearly on questions of moral theology and sexual ethics.

Many countries need to look afresh at their Christian roots and long-held Christian beliefs and traditions. Much has been forgotten, and much that was once regarded as part of the average person's knowledge in the fields of the Bible and Christian teaching is now unknown to the average person. This knowledge needs to be learned once more and the church should be the teacher both by direct means of teaching in schools and churches and by such indirect means as radio and television.

Christians as servants

Individuals and institutions which are part of the church have traditionally nursed in times of plague. In particular, convents and monasteries had a caring and nursing role for many centuries. Some of these convents now have a teaching function, many of them being boarding schools for two or three hundred residents. As the epidemic progresses, some monasteries and convents may feel a call to take up again the role of nursing and caring for the sick.

Recently a twelve-bedded ward was opened in a London hospital to care for people with AIDS. If this ward were to be used for a hospice role, it could accommodate no more than eighty-four people a year, because experience in San Francisco has shown that an average of forty-seven days is needed for each person dying with AIDS. This gives a bed availability of seven patients per bed per year.

Now set that against a convent with three hundred beds. Such a resource would enable 2,100 people to be cared for in the same length of time. There is time to prepare for this by prayerful planning and training of individual nuns, monks and others in hospice caring. After all, the whole hospice movement for care of the terminally ill has been suffused with Christian insights and involvement. If the epidemic increases to levels such as those seen in the United States and Africa, this will become one of the church's most vital roles.

The general population will be deeply distressed by the epidemic, which will affect many of its younger people. Christians will have a role of comforter, caring for the many who will have lost their 'comfort in old age', their children.

An international force

The church is an international community, with more members in the developing world than in the West. The work in such regions takes many forms— medical care, education, support of specific development projects, language translation, church planting and nourishing. The AIDS epidemic will come to affect people working in all of these areas. But much more importantly, those who are working in these areas can affect the AIDS epidemic. They can have a tremendous effect on the future of the community which they are serving, and can make the difference between the people surviving and thriving for the future generations, or dying.

Workers do not have to be medically qualified to have an enormous impact on the AIDS situation wherever they go, as it is education which is needed in order to enable those who are not infected to survive, and basic nursing skills can easily be taught to enable the dying to be cared for in greater dignity and comfort. Christian workers in developing countries, both nationals and expatriates, can contribute more now than at any other time, for this is the time of the greatest need in these regions.

A Christian is bringing good news at a time of great need. The news is a message of hope, of God and his guidelines and this is a message which has never been more relevant to people's lives.

5

How Far Will AIDS Spread?

It is hard for most people to take on board the full seriousness of the AIDS epidemic. We are now at the stage when the epidemic is beginning to gather momentum, but so far the numbers dying are not so great as those from some other major diseases. The full impact is yet to come, as more and more people become infected with HIV, and those already infected develop AIDS and die.

The disease has already spread widely, and it is going to spread further. But how far will it spread?

Early in 1986 it was estimated that worldwide there were 100,000 people with AIDS, 300,000 to 500,000 persons with other symptoms of HIV infection, and between 5 and 10 million people infected with HIV but not showing any symptoms. The World Health Organization estimate that by 1991 there will be between 50 and 100 million infected with HIV. As the numbers infected continue to double every six months to a year, the rapid increase in infection on a global scale can readily be appreciated.

Just to give a small example, in Kampala, Uganda, pregnant women were tested on attending an antenatal booking clinic. In October 1985, 107 were tested and 10.7 per cent found HIV-positive.

Between February and April 1986, 1,000 tested gave 13.5 per cent positive. And out of 170 tested in February 1987, 24.1 per cent were positive.

The rapid increase is a consequence of the fact that AIDS results from a virus infection, one person can give it to two people, two people to four, four to eight and so on. The longer a person lives, the more people he or she can infect, the more rapidly the disease spreads and the more people die in the end. And remember that a person with HIV can live free of symptoms for many months or years.

The rapid increase in infection is also a consequence of the enormous increase in urbanization. The *urban* population of the world today is equivalent to the *total* world population in 1950. In every country both HIV infection and AIDS are more common in cities than in rural areas.

It has also been shown that the numbers of those infected can be pushed up dramatically by a relatively small number of people each of whom has a high number of sexual contacts. This seems to have happened in the homosexual community in San Francisco and among some heterosexual males in Africa. It also applies, of course, to prostitutes.

The AIDS iceberg

It has been estimated that for every known case of AIDS there may be as many as 50 to a 100 infected individuals, most of whom will have no symptoms. This means that by the time five people show signs of AIDS in a city, 500 are likely to have been infected with HIV. By the time those five people have died of

AIDS, between 2,000—3,000 will have been infected with HIV.

In San Francisco 24,000 out of 100,000 of the homosexual population were infected with HIV before the first case of AIDS there was identified. Because of the long period of time between infection and developing AIDS a large number of people may have become infected before the community is alerted to the danger. The chart on page 43 shows how the epidemic in the United States progressed.

It should be remembered that in this new epidemic knowledge about the pattern of spread of HIV is still limited. While it is certain that the number of AIDS cases is increasing rapidly, we do not yet know the answers to some important questions about its spread in the future.

This makes precise predictions extremely difficult. Looking at the predicted numbers of new AIDS cases in Britain for the years 1985-88, from which the government and health departments have been working, we see a predicted figure given, but widely divergent figures above and below it are also given to show the range within which there is ninety-five per cent certainty that the actual figure will fall. In their evidence to the Government Select Committee, the Terrence Higgins Trust warned that two million people may be infected by 1991.

There are several factors which make predictions difficult:

● **Will the virus mutate (change its form)?** This remains an unknown quantity, although it has already appeared in more than one form. If a mutation occurs which affects its mode of transmission, this may affect the routes it will take and the speed of its spread. In any case the ability to mutate poses major problems in finding either a cure or a vaccine. The future rate of spread of the virus is difficult to predict. It may be a slower rate, or it may become a faster one, depending on factors as yet unknown.

● **How far will AIDS spread to the heterosexual population?** Worldwide, two different patterns of HIV infection have emerged. Pattern 1 is where HIV is found first in haemophiliacs, blood-transfusion patients, male homosexuals, and intravenous drug abusers. This characterizes HIV's progress in the United States, Europe and parts of Asia and Latin America. Pattern 2 is where HIV is found mainly in sexually active adults of either sex, as in Central, East and Southern Africa.

There are now strong indications that countries which started with pattern 1 will eventually move into pattern 2. This has already happened in Haiti, and concern is growing sharply that Haiti's transition is being followed in North America and Europe.

If this transition does take place, the numbers dying will move rapidly upwards. Recently an Edinburgh professor of Actuarial Science (the science of statistical predictions) did a study for an insurance company of the likely figures for AIDS in Britain by the late 1990s. He assumed only a low risk for heterosexuals but that all those who expose themselves to high-risk factors will become infected and die. On this basis he predicted an annual death toll rising to 48,000 in Britain by 1998, after which the

AIDS Growth in the United States

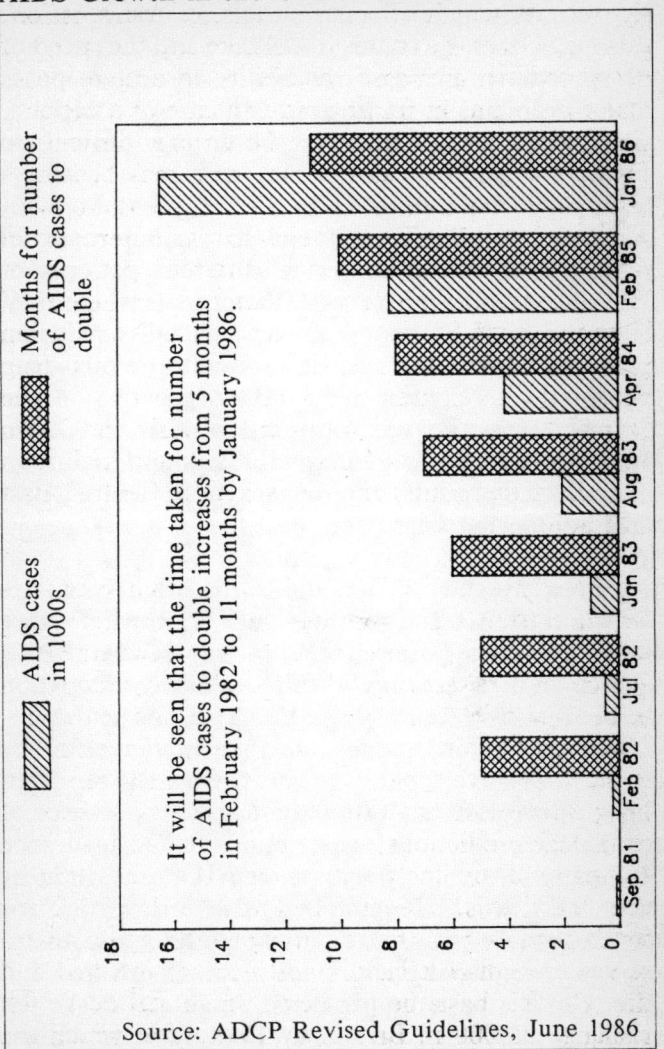

Months for number of AIDS cases to double

AIDS cases in 1000s

It will be seen that the time taken for number of AIDS cases to double increases from 5 months in February 1982 to 11 months by January 1986.

Source: ADCP Revised Guidelines, June 1986

figures would level out, although AIDS would present a serious health problem for another forty years. But what if his initial assumption is wrong, and the virus does move across to heterosexuals in a major way? Then his figures would prove much too low.

It has been suggested that this spread into the heterosexual population is not happening as fast as expected. There are several reasons why this may be so. The development of AIDS takes time, and the proportion of heterosexuals with AIDS in Europe and the United States represents only the picture of the epidemic between three and five years ago, when few heterosexuals were infected with HIV. We do not know who or where most of those infected with HIV are. Only 6,000 seropositive people are informally reported out of a possible 100,000 people infected with HIV in Britain.

● **What proportion of those with HIV will develop AIDS?** It is now thought that the median incubation period from infection with HIV to developing AIDS is between five and eight years. This means that the virus can spread widely and silently within the population before many of those infected with HIV show symptoms and signs of AIDS.

Only recently research seemed to show that between twenty and thirty per cent of people infected with HIV would develop AIDS within three years, while a further thirty per cent would have symptoms. But as the months go by, the situation looks worse. A study in Frankfurt published in August 1986 showed that out of 377 HIV carriers followed up, only thirty

How AIDS May Grow

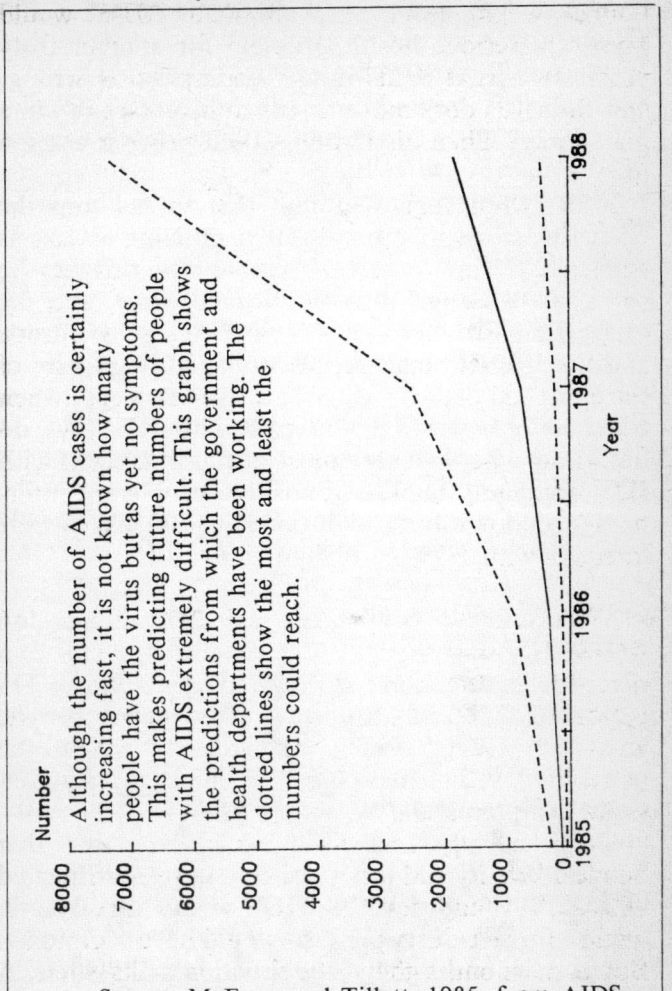

Although the number of AIDS cases is certainly increasing fast, it is not known how many people have the virus but as yet no symptoms. This makes predicting future numbers of people with AIDS extremely difficult. This graph shows the predictions from which the government and health departments have been working. The dotted lines show the most and least the numbers could reach.

Source: McEvoy and Tillett, 1985, from <u>AIDS - Forecasting its Impact, OHE.</u>

remained symptom-free. It is now forecasted that seventy-five per cent of carriers will develop AIDS within seven years. Many experts believe that everyone infected with HIV will eventually develop AIDS. Obviously this is another factor likely to push up the figures radically.

● **How readily will people change their lifestyles?** Will the government education programmes persuade people at risk to make radical changes to eliminate or reduce the risk of infection? The sector of society with most responsibility, the government, found it difficult to grasp the reality of the danger of the AIDS epidemic for three, perhaps four years. (Hence the silence I found so puzzling in 1985.) It would not be surprising, therefore, if the younger generation found it difficult to grasp the reality of the danger of the epidemic for another three years. It takes time to change attitudes and lifestyles. But maybe this is too pessimistic. Perhaps there will be a greater readiness among young people to adapt to change.

It would appear that new cases of venereal disease have dropped dramatically in homosexual males. This would imply that risky sexual behaviour has been dramatically reduced. However, if the number of new cases of venereal disease has halved while the incidence of HIV infection in a population has quadrupled, that still leaves an ever-increasing risk of HIV infection in those who do maintain risky lifestyles. Data which appears to show evidence of changes of behaviour should be interpreted with caution.

Education does not stop the epidemic, it merely

slows the spread. If we wait until we know all the answers then we will wait until it is too late to influence the course of the epidemic. It is far better to take steps that may with hindsight prove unnecessary, than to wait until it is too late. The facts available are the only ones we have, and these we must use.

● **If people use condoms, will that stop AIDS spreading?** For those who are not leading a lifestyle which gives total safety from infection, it is important that they take such measures as are possible to reduce their risk of infection. The regular, consistent and correct use of condoms, preferably with a water-based spermicide, has been recommended as dramatically lowering, though not altogether removing, the risk of HIV infection.

However, condoms are by no means a totally reliable protection. For one thing, not all condoms are perfect. A recent survey by *Self Health* magazine showed significant failure rates, more in some brands than others. Also, condoms have to be correctly used every time.

Perhaps for these reasons, pregnancies do occasionally occur, and a recent study showed that between thirteen and fifteen per cent of women whose husbands used the sheath as their sole means of contraception became pregnant within one year. This failure rate is unacceptable for a sheath used for contraceptive purposes, but much more so if it is the sole means of protecting us from a fatal infection. And pregnancy can only occur on certain days in a woman's cycle, while HIV infection can be transmitted at any time.

All this boils down to saying that to trust in condoms to protect us from AIDS is like playing Russian roulette. It makes infection less likely, but a person persisting with a risky lifestyle over a significant period is still in grave danger of infection even if condoms are used.

6

The One Sure Defence

Because this new epidemic is a disease which is spread mainly through sexual contact, it is in part a personal private disease. But it is also a disease of wider public importance.

Patterns of behaviour involving sex need to be examined, including courting patterns and marriage patterns, and homosexual sex. When talking about these we are really talking about *people*, individuals with hopes and disappointments, joys and sorrows, longings for companionship and fears of rejection.

But situations and behaviour may change, particularly when danger threatens, and personal changes may need to be made as a response to AIDS.

A new era of sexuality

The biblical writer of Proverbs composed this poem more than 3,000 years ago. Yet it beautifully captures the approach to sexual relationships we need to find again today.

> Find joy with the wife you
> married in your youth,
> fair as a hind,
> graceful as a fawn.
> Let hers be the company you keep,

hers the breasts that ever
fill you with delight,
hers the love that ever
holds you captive.

Sometimes the 'AIDS scare' is depicted as restricting people's enjoyment of sex, as if it were being said, 'You can't enjoy yourselves; you have to be careful.'

And indeed monogamous sex is perceived as boring by many people. But this is very far from being true, and in the new era it will be the only interesting exciting sex! For it is the only context in which one will be able to avoid the paraphernalia of spermicides and condoms, and the ever-present anxiety that the virus will nevertheless get through by some accident. This is quite apart from all the other benefits of monogamy such as emotional stability and the joy of life within a family.

Claire Rayner has some perceptive words about monogamy in her recent book *Safe Sex*.

'It is not necessarily true that a person who chooses to share all his or her sex with one individual is a bore; to suggest that is to say that the only part of a person's anatomy that matters is the genitals, and that unless they are leaping from bed to bed, exercising said genitals vigorously with all sorts of different people, their brains are atrophying. In my experience the reverse is true . . .

'It is far from romantic flimflam to say that the happiest lives are likely to be built on a relationship that has moved from slow and gentle courtship, taking each sexual step one at a time and slowly, rather than in the all-at-once bound that has been fashionable for the past few years, to permanent commitment sealed with a public statement of some kind (a wedding, in other words) . . .

'That is why a lot of people are going to opt for lifelong monogamy as a lifestyle, because they have realized that not only does it protect them from nasty diseases that can and do shorten life; it can also be fun and comfortable and make you feel secure.'

Many of today's young people are very far from promiscuous. 'Serial monogamy' is now an accepted pattern of courting behaviour for many. This means that an unmarried person is 'faithful' to his or her partner until that relationship ends and is replaced by another sexual partnership.

But in terms of openness to HIV infection serial monogamy is by no means a safe lifestyle. If a young man or woman has eight sexual partners before marriage, and they have each had eight sexual partners, then by just counting chains of two links of sexual partners there may be as many as 500 contacts, and potentially 500 chances of becoming linked with HIV. Serial monogamy is potentially a killer.

Protective friendship

The kind of sex which says, 'What can I have?', rather than 'What can I give?' is like a drug. Having indulged, you know exactly what you are missing, and this explains why abstinence is so much more difficult following the first enjoyable act of inter-course. How can we return to the world of two generations ago in which it was the norm for girls to say 'No', in the sense of 'not yet'?

The myth must be destroyed that it is a recipe for disaster to marry without 'first trying him or her out in bed'. It is this myth which leads to the pheno-menon of serial monogamy. Then we must re-learn the 'Two Rs' of Respect and Romance. It is surely not unrealistic to try and rediscover for this genera-tion that the sex part of their body and psyche is precious and special, not for throwing around. 'Petting' will need to become 'enough for just now', though eventually a prelude to far better lovemaking (within marriage or its equivalent) than the modern rushed job.

Another important message is that, even if one is no longer a virgin, there are still many advantages in becoming chaste, from now until we discover our eventual life partner.

A valuable idea is that of 'protective friendship'. This concept looks towards the future and the well-being and safety of the girlfriend or boyfriend. Courting does not include sexual intercourse as this would establish in the two individuals a sexual pattern of courting for the future. Although that particular partnership would have had no risk of catching HIV infection, the future safety of the loved one is all-important. If the friendship does not actually lead to marriage, then it will have provided a safe bridge for those two people to bring them nearer in time to the safety of a faithful monogamous partnership.

As the chart on page 55 shows, there are two types of sexual partnership. In one type, two persons enjoy sexual experience only with each other. These individuals have no risk of getting AIDS, nor any other sexually transmitted disease.

The other type involves multiple sexual partnerships, which permit the spread of HIV. Both partners here have a risk of infection because they have become linked to a network of other partners, even though they are not highly promiscous.

It is not easy to stick to one partner for life. But the inclination to participate in unwise sexual relationships is not fundamentally different from the inclination to spend money you don't have, or to eat or drink more than is good for you. And there is help available. This help is called marriage, and marriage has many benefits:

● **Marriage is something to look forward to.** Saving sex until you are married is not very different from saving money in a bank. Both require that we forgo an immediate pleasure for the sake of a better pleasure later on. It is difficult to think of anything potentially more ruinous to sexual pleasure than the fear of getting AIDS.

● **Marriage helps people to maintain their mutual commitment to an exclusive sexual partnership.** It provides a relationship of mutual dependency and help.

● **And lifelong, exclusive partnerships can be the most rewarding way to have sex.** An ancient sex manual called the Song of Songs shows that enjoying sex is a matter of adapting to and learning about your partner. This requires trust—something that is marred by multiple partnerships. Another ancient way of putting it is that marriage is two people becoming one person—emotionally, spiritually and physically.

Some people worry that it is too late to adopt such a lifestyle. But they need not worry. The virus has not yet spread extensively beyond homosexual men and those who abuse intravenous drugs. The vast majority of people can remain free of any risk of infection if they begin now to maintain exclusive partnerships.

Education in relationships

We have said that we need to return to Christian teaching. But Christian teaching in the area of sex can seem always to be negative. It also has generally followed the world in being far too concerned with genital activity, whereas sex is really about mutual relationship, or, in a word, love. Dr Jack Dominian argues that the fundamental feature of sex is its powerful role in pair-bonding. This creates its own appetite for more of the same and produces its own ethic with an almost inevitable momentum towards permanence and exclusiveness. Having many sexual partners is not just undesirable because it is dangerous: it is wrong because it is disordered, out of line with the way God made us. The bonding functions of sex were not invented by psychiatrists but by God.

This is very important in sex education, which with the advent of AIDS is a new part of health education. Young people will not listen to a point-

The Sexual Spread of HIV

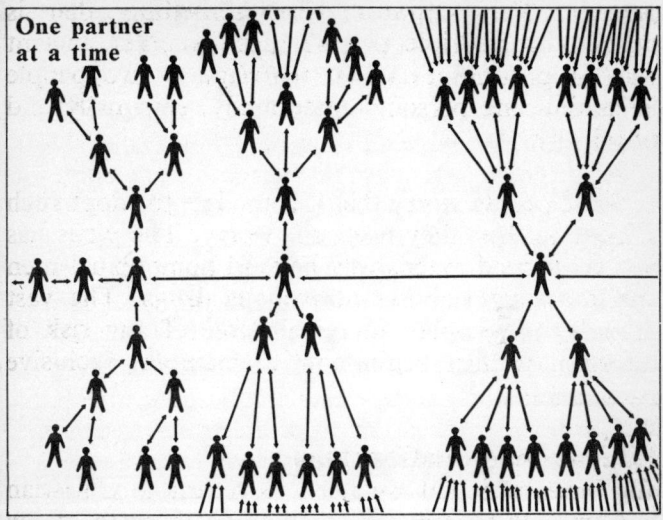

One partner at a time

By the eighth partner in the series, the range of contacts reaches 500, if both partners have the same lifestyle.

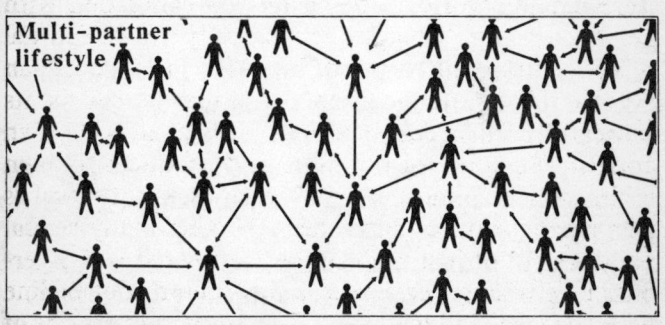

Multi-partner lifestyle

More risky contacts than can fit on this page.

One partner for life — No chance of infection.

blank 'No'. But they will at least consider the word 'Wait', if its advantages are well argued. The preventive messages about AIDS (celibacy, monogamy, use a condom) seem so negative, anti-fun, dull if not totally unreasonable. To quote Dr Malcolm Potts, those at greatest risk are in their late teens and early twenties, 'who are both the most sexually active and often believe themselves immortal. Risk-taking and AIDS are not unlike risk-taking and pregnancy—neither AIDS infection nor fertilization are certain, the gambler often survives, and the penalty is remote—at least nine months in the case of pregnancy and maybe years in the case of AIDS'.

For health education to work it must convince young people of three things:

- They are at risk;
- A lethal disease may reveal no symptoms;
- 'Safer sex' offers worthwhile protection.

The battle will be lost if any link in this chain is broken. 'One thing is certain,' writes Dr Potts, 'success in the control of the AIDS epidemic will turn on the same respect and concern for individuals which has characterized successful family planning services.'

A helpful illustration comes in the book *I Married You*, in which the author compares sexual intercourse to the glue between two pieces of paper: 'If you try to separate two pieces of paper which are glued together, you tear them both. If you try to separate a couple who cleave together, both are hurt.' Multiple partners means multiple 'bust-ups', which are bound to cause emotional hurt, or hardness as a protective reaction. This in turn makes it more difficult to develop with any future partner the mutual trust which is the cornerstone of a secure home for children.

If more people restrict sexual experience to one lifelong partnership, this has a population effect which is like herd immunity in infectious diseases. It means that potential networks are broken in numerous places and the transmission of an agent like HIV is less likely. Monogamous behaviour by one partner makes monogamous behaviour by the other more likely. An exclusive bond consists of psychological and emotional as well as physical strands. Marriage hedges sex about with financial and social considerations. The public education campaign concerning AIDS so far has neglected the unique features and qualitative distinction of monogamous marriage.

So far governments have carefully avoided advertising the means by which the spread of HIV can be brought under control. The complete absence of any mention of marriage in literature produced by a statutory body must mean hostility, ignorance or political fear. Perhaps this is further testimony of the extent to which the electorate has become alienated from Christianity. The safe-sex campaign at least recognizes that sexual activity is part of the normal routine of life for most people. Celibacy is no answer to AIDS from a population standpoint. The natural implication is that as far as the government is concerned marriage is a more dangerous subject than AIDS.

There is a yet more fundamental dilemma,

however. Human beings do not easily change their behaviour. They will clutch at less painful solutions. Any physician who has attempted to get patients to lose weight will be familiar with this propensity. Advocacy of safe sex and the possibilities of an HIV vaccine undermine the obvious lesson from AIDS that changes in sexual behaviour and in attitudes toward marriage must occur. There is no doubt that AIDS has concentrated the minds of many people concerning sexual behaviour. It is indeed ironic that the activities of the government impair this process. Safe sex and vaccine research have nothing to do with compassion towards those already infected with HIV or suffering with AIDS. They are half-baked public health approaches that have been dictated by fear of public opinion.

Would it not be preferable for government-sponsored education programmes on AIDS to be sufficiently direct and uncompromising to measure up to the true scale of the problem? This has been expressed, as it relates particularly to developing countries, by Dr Jonathan Mann, Director of the Special Programme on AIDS:

> The major social impact of AIDS worldwide is the direct result of the dominant role of sexual transmission of HIV. But, the brunt of illness and death is currently borne by the twenty to forty-nine year olds. In contrast to many public health problems which slectively affect either the very young or the old, AIDS affects the most vital segment of the population in terms of social or economic development. The selective involvement

of young and middle-aged adults—including
business and government cadres and members of
social, economic and political élites—leads to
potential for economic and political destabilization
in areas of the developing world most severely
affected by HIV. What political system could with-
stand the ultimate destabilizing impact of a twenty
or twenty-five per cent or higher HIV-infection
rate among young adults?

7

The God Dimension

Some people maintain that AIDS is not a moral issue, and certainly not a religious one. The churches, they say, should mind their own spiritual business and allow medical technicians to progress towards the solution of a problem which is essentially medical, not ethical, in nature.

Simply to state that view is to expose its weaknesses. The most urgent issue facing us today concerns the spread of HIV. With a few exceptions, HIV spreads through well-defined behaviour patterns, rooted in chosen lifestyles. Ethics and morality are, by definition, to do with the choices people make in setting the direction of their lives and with their day-to-day behaviour. It is therefore short-sighted to see no link between the need to control this particular disease and the corresponding need to think deeply and radically about the behaviour which spreads it.

And if morality is relevant, so is religion. The Christian gospel does not address disembodied souls. The Bible teaches that God created us to live in a certain way, and both New and Old Testaments set out ideals for human behaviour as well as guidelines for committed Christian living. If an atheist says, 'These ideals are irrelevant to me, because I do not believe in the existence of a Creator,' the Bible replies, 'You are wrong. Those ideals are inescapably relevant, because you are made in the image of the God you do not believe in.' In other words God created human beings, not Christians only. And his laws are framed for the well-being of the whole human race without distinction. The claim that some behaviour patterns lead to human health and happiness while others do not—simply because of the way people are made—surely merits a hearing from a generation which faces the global threat of AIDS. Perhaps this lay behind the embarrassment of an anonymous psychologist who cares for many AIDS patients, when he was asked by a journalist, 'If we had played by New Testament rules on sexual behaviour, would we have ever had an epidemic?' 'Of course not,' he replied, 'but, for God's sake, don't quote me on that!'

There are three false contrasts that often stop people thinking clearly about the moral and spiritual dimension to the AIDS threat.

Rules and results

Anyone who criticizes the kind of behaviour which encourages the spread of HIV is liable to be charged with 'moralizing', with overtones of legalism and unjustified interference in the lives of others. Alternative approaches which major on preventive measures ('safe sex') are exempt from this charge, because they do not appear to make moral judgments on what other people do.

But this is false contrast number one. On both sides of the argument there is an attempt to show that some practices (unprotected anal intercourse, for example, and the sharing of hypodermic needles) are to be discouraged. Those who refuse to label anything as wrong in itself are still drawing moral distinctions and making moral judgments when they discourage the kind of behaviour which results in more people getting AIDS now. They are still doing their best to persuade others, 'You ought not to behave in this or that particular way at the present time.'

The difference, of course, lies in the routes taken to arrive at the common conclusion. Opponents of 'moralizing' insist that sexual conduct is value-free. A particular practice only becomes wrong, they say, when its results are overwhelmingly bad. It is wrong, therefore, to have anal intercourse so long as that practice carries a high risk of spreading a lethal disease. If, at some time in the future, the risk is nullified, anal intercourse may become right once again in certain circumstances.

But if we believe there are certain unchangeable rules, then we take a different route. Following our ethical code, with its principles and rules for behaviour, we insist that particular forms of behaviour are wrong in themselves, whatever the consequences that follow.

In the debate about AIDS it is often assumed that Christians and other religious people follow the rules route, while everybody else makes moral judgments on the basis of results. That, however, is not quite true.

Christians certainly have principles and rules (God-given, they believe) to direct their behaviour.

Among them are the biblical vetoes on homosexual acts and sex outside marriage. But the Bible also encourages believers to modify the way they behave by thinking about the long-term consequences of certain lifestyles. As the apostle Paul put it in a nutshell, 'A man reaps what he sows.'

'Long-term' is the operative word. People who make their judgments between right and wrong by measuring consequences can only take into account the results they foresee. Inevitably, such horizons are limited. Who foresaw AIDS in the 1960s? The Bible, on the other hand, declares the *eventual* results of certain behaviour patterns. The authority of its predictions rests (Christians believe) on the reputation of the best Long-Range Forecaster in the business. God sees over all human horizons. So when the New Testament declares that all extra-marital intercourse leads to human disaster, the Christian takes the forecast seriously, even when the exact shape of the consequences is lost in the mists of the future.

The arrival of AIDS fills Christians with intense sadness, but it does not take them by surprise, because the relationship of rules to results is that of signpost to destination. The warning signals along the road have been there for centuries. It is only those who refuse to read the writing who are shocked by the appearance of cosmic disaster round the next bend. And, Christians want to add, even when the medical solution to AIDS is found (and may it be soon) the road will only lead on to further human unhappiness of a different, unforeseen kind. Why not start keeping the rules now, they ask, and pay sensible attention to the signposts?

Public and private

Ten years before the Sexual Offences Act (which decriminalized homosexual acts between consenting adults in private) became effective in Britain, the Wolfenden Committee had paved the way by drawing a sharp distinction between public and private behaviour. Wolfenden argued that it was not 'proper for the law to concern itself with what a man does in private unless it can be shown to be so contrary to the public good that the law ought to intervene in its function as the guardian of that public good'.

The distinction itself was not at all new. John Stuart Mill had articulated it very powerfully in his famous tract *On Liberty* in 1859. 'The only purpose for which power can be rightfully exercised over any member of a civilized community, against his will,' he wrote, 'is to prevent harm to others.'

This plea for personal liberty swayed Members of Parliament in 1967. Men over twenty-one who wished to practise anal intercourse in private, they concluded, should no longer have to do so with the threat of the law hanging over their heads.

The arrival of AIDS has set a large question mark beside that conclusion. When over eighty-five per cent of known cases in Britain arise within the homosexual community, and when experience in Africa and the United States indicates that the heterosexual majority will not remain safe for long (through intravenous addicts, contaminated blood products and bisexual intercourse), it can no longer be argued that an act of anal intercourse is of no interest to anyone but the couple concerned. The boundary between private and public has been blurred.

AIDS is very much a personal *and* a public concern. What one person does by way of risking the spread of HIV has far-reaching consequences for others unknown to him or her. Society as a whole, therefore, must take on the responsibility for influencing individual behaviour.

Legal penalties would be hard to enforce as a deterrent, though the time may well come when the movement of AIDS victims has to be monitored or even restricted—by coercion if necessary. In the meantime, carrots are probably more effective than sticks. The provision, at public expense, of free condoms for those who continue to put themselves at risk sexually, and of clean needles for those who cannot or will not break free from drug abuse, is the price society must pay for safeguarding the health of the majority. So is a government-sponsored advertising campaign which is openly aimed at persuading individuals to change their freely chosen habits.

If this erosion of personal liberty makes us uneasy, we should remember how readily we accept similar controls in other areas of life. We limit freedom of speech by laws against libel, and no one complains. We curb acts of racial discrimination, and all fair-minded people applaud. Such laws actually promote freedom by restricting it. We censor the atmosphere by creating smokeless zones—so the majority can breathe more freely. We even have laws to limit noises and smells—in the interests of public health. It is only an extension of this principle to seek to discourage any behaviour which risks the well-being of the majority. Christians would want to add that genuine liberty is only to be found when the individual's will is submitted to the law of God as well as of governments. Released from behaviour patterns which dehumanize their victims, men and women experience the refreshing liberty of relating to others as their Maker always intended.

Condemnation and compassion

AIDS is not God's judgment on every single individual who catches it. That is a caricature of God, making him out to be a capricious Creator who aims the thunderbolts of his punishment with a careless disregard for justice. Why do haemophiliacs become infected? Why do wives of unfaithful husbands die of the disease, along with their babies? Why do male homosexuals run such dreadful risks, while most lesbians escape? Those who imply that every individual who contracts AIDS is being directly punished by God for his or her personal sins have no acceptable answers to these questions.

Christians do, however, see in the AIDS epidemic the hand of God's judgment on a corrupt *society*. The New Testament warns very plainly that people who tear up the Creator's blueprint must live and die with the consequences. Those who give up God and his values inevitably experience the results of losing the social protection of his norms. We live in a society which encourages behaviour that leads directly to the spread of AIDS. It follows that those who catch it are the victims not only of a lethal virus but of a society which dresses up as normal patterns of behaviour which God condemns.

Even this limited relationship of God's judgment with AIDS, however, appears 'judgmental' to some people. Surely, they protest, Jesus would want us to treat AIDS sufferers with bold compassion. There is, of course, an important truth here. We cannot ignore the way Jesus exposed the hypocrisy of religious people who were so preoccupied with picking splinters out of other people's eyes that they completely failed to notice the huge planks of wood in their own. Time and time again, the Gospel writers tell us how he was 'moved with compassion' by human need, whether or not the sufferers had brought their fate on themselves. He would undoubtedly have beaten the Minister of Health to the first handshake in an AIDS ward.

But there is another side to the truth which is equally important. Jesus exposed sin with such candour that his life was soon at risk. He saw no contradiction at all between warm compassion and piercing criticism. When a woman was brought to him after being caught in the act of adultery, he told her to change her lifestyle with that same simple frankness which made her accusers creep away in shame.

It is not, in fact, at all compassionate to withhold correction in the name of love. Men and women who get caught up with the abuse of drugs or sex (and thus run an above-average risk of catching and spreading AIDS) face temptations which become increasingly difficult to fight off. Their only hope of change lies in being convinced that change is essential. The battles will never be won unless people are sure the war is worth fighting.

The Christian would want to add the tail-piece that it is possible to break habits and alter deeply ingrained lifestyles. The most important thing the Christian gospel has to offer anyone in need is the promise of fresh, effective, supernatural resources to achieve change.

8

To Test or Not to Test

One vital question to do with the containment of AIDS has become highly contentious. Should people be tested for HIV? This is partly a question of public policy, but it is also a pressing personal question for many. Should I have an HIV test, if I have been involved in a risky lifestyle?

First of all, what does this test involve?

Different tests for HIV

There are several methods of testing currently in use, the most reliable of which is complicated and expensive. What follows is simply a brief summary of a complex medical field.

The ELISA test, which stands for enzyme-linked immunosorbent assay, is the easiest and cheapest test widely used and takes between two and five hours to complete, costing fifty pence. The Dupont dipstick test takes forty-five minutes and costs £2. The latest 'Matchbox test' uses a drop of blood and takes only five minutes. If a test is positive for HIV it is repeated and then confirmed by a different type of test. Because it may take a few weeks before antibodies are produced, any blood test may need to be repeated, even if it is negative at the first go.

Delayed seroconversion (a delay in the blood

becoming positive to one of these tests) may result in false reassurance. There is a vital need to make cheaply available a viral antigen test, to add to the range of tests already in use.

This is so that in the first few weeks of infection, when antibodies to HIV are not yet produced, the presence of the virus in the blood can be identified. But it must be emphasized that a reliable antigen test is not yet available.

Personal and social factors

Early in the epidemic there was a heavy bias towards advising people who thought they might have become infected, *not* to have the HIV antibody test. There were several reasons for this. When the blood test became available in 1985, the majority of those infected were homosexual men in America. They quickly realized that if they were diagnosed as HIV-antibody-positive this would mean that those who did not already have health insurance would be unlikely to obtain it. Without health insurance, a serious illness could mean major hospital bills and sometimes destitution. For a large proportion of American working men, health insurance was paid for by the employing firm. Loss of employment would therefore mean loss of health insurance with all that this entailed.

At the time when testing for antibody to HIV became available, it was thought that only ten per cent of those who were infected would eventually develop AIDS. A positive test was therefore thought to mean only that a person had a one in ten chance of developing the disease. It was thought that to know one was HIV-positive would arouse unnecessary anxieties. But now, as has already been pointed out, the known and projected figures for people with HIV going on to develop AIDS are much higher, and many experts believe the majority will eventually develop the disease. So the situation has changed.

There are several compelling reasons why people at risk should be tested:

● **To stop infected people spreading the virus**
Early in the epidemic the emphasis was put on protecting those who were known to be HIV-positive or with AIDS. Now it is increasingly being realized that there is another responsibility: to protect those not yet infected. With rare exceptions, a person who knows that he or she is infected is likely to be strongly motivated to protect those nearest and dearest to him from infection. It is very much to the practical advantage of the infected person that those who might be helpful to him or her do not acquire a fatal disease. This is in addition to the altruistic desire to protect those whom one loves. The HIV antibody test, confirmed by other tests, enables a person to know for certain whether they are infected.

It is difficult to change lifestyles, and by and large people only acquire the motivation to do so when they have been tested. Though this is chiefly so if the result is positive, a negative result may also be beneficial—just as negative pregnancy tests after a scare have been known to increase people's motivation to use contraception. Although the implications for lifestyle are therefore the same whatever the result, people's capacity for wishful thinking is so great that they are likely to carry on in the same old way unless the test is actually done.

In many respects being found to be HIV-positive presents the same devastating implications as the diagnosis of any other potentially fatal illness. The problem is not so much the particular nature of AIDS as the fact that it is potentially fatal. A person with a fatal illness is unlikely to be able to obtain life insurance or an endowment mortgage. However never in the past has this meant that a doctor discourages a person from having investigations to diagnose a fatal condition, especially one with such enormous public health implications, to preserve an individual's economic status.

If a single HIV-positive person is not tested, and persists with the same sexual or needle-sharing life-style, it is perfectly possible for him to infect up to three figures of other people with HIV as a consequence in, say, five years time—avoidable cases, if the first person had avoided passing on the infection after being found positive. By making tests difficult to come by, or by counselling against having the test done, we are all behaving as though the deaths of dozens of people in a few years' time are less important than one individual's present-day rights in regard to getting a mortgage. It is not inconsistent with real sympathy for people who receive a virtual death sentence to say that the rights of today's individuals must be balanced against those of many more people down the line in five to ten years' time. If only fifty people are infected with HIV for each person with AIDS, by the time they themselves have developed AIDS fifty times fifty, that is 2,500, are infected from the original source.

● **To guard against infected women becoming pregnant** Now that HIV infection is spreading into the heterosexual population, women are becoming infected. It is important for an HIV-positive woman to know that she is infected, as this will affect not only her future lifestyle, but also whether or not she becomes pregnant. This is for two reasons. First, any babies born to her have a very great risk of being born infected and dying of AIDS. Second, pregnancy in an HIV-positive woman is thought to produce full-blown AIDS earlier than would otherwise occur, and she may die years before she would otherwise have done. If she already has a family, this possibility assumes even greater significance.

● **To help people with AIDS take action early when symptoms begin** This is another reason why it is to the HIV-positive person's advantage to know their HIV status. Seventy-five per cent of people presenting with AIDS present with a life-threatening illness, half of these a chest infection. For an HIV-positive person therefore a chest infection is very important, as it may be the onset of pneumocystis carinii pneumonia. If this diagnosis is not made, and correct treatment for this rare condition not started, that person will probably die. To know that one is HIV-positive therefore makes the likelihood of longer survival greater.

● **To give the possibility of slowing the progress of the illness** It is commonly stated that, as there is no cure and no treatment, it is of no benefit to know if one is HIV-positive. This statement may well be out-of-date, as research is developing less toxic drugs to slow the multiplication of the virus. At first only people with AIDS received treatment with drugs such as AZT in high doses and, for many, with highly toxic side effects.

In his lecture at the Royal College of Physicians, Robert Gallo expressed the opinion that instead of starting treatment when a person's immune system is severely damaged and full-blown AIDS present, people should receive low-dose treatment at a much earlier stage to prevent or reduce further damage to the immune system. Trials of AZT on seropositive people are planned by the Medical Research Council and some trial treatments are in progress. It is important that people know their HIV status so that as treatment becomes available to slow the progressive HIV damage, the people who can benefit from it are identified.

However it is suspiciously true that an area of unidentified need costs nothing to meet. (For instance, the annual cost of treating 50,000 people with only a fifth of the daily dose of AZT now used would be £50 million.) There may be some in positions of power who have a vested interest in not discovering the precise size of the seropositive pool because of the high cost of treatment. This should not be a reason for not identifying the seropositivity of those infected.

9

Can AIDS Be Contained?

So far we have shown enough to make it clear that AIDS poses a greater threat than most people realize: as big a threat to the at-risk generation as the plagues of earlier times. We have seen that, although many people have taken from government advertising the message 'Use condoms to be safe', in fact the only safe sex now is with one partner for life.

But what if many people do not change their lifestyle? What could the implications be?

In this final chapter we review what governments are doing, and go on to assess the likely course of the epidemic in Britain and the probable cost in economic and human terms. But all this is intended to make us look squarely at the options that face us. And we end with some specific proposals for action.

What governments are doing
Most governments have programmes of some kind to combat AIDS. The United States spent $340 million in 1986 on research alone. The British government is to allocate £50 million for the year 1988 to cope with the rising cost of the disease. The programme of the British Government may serve as an illustration of the attempts developed countries are making in face of the crisis.

● **Research is being sponsored.** Increasing amounts of money are being allocated for research into AIDS. Over twenty projects are approved for support by the Medical Research Council, at a cost of £2.4 million. A further £1 million a year for AIDS research has been allocated from 1987–88. The government has made a total of £14.5 million additional aid available to the Medical Research Council between 1987 and 1990. This research is aimed at finding a vaccine to prevent AIDS, and to develop antiviral drugs.

The Medical Research Council co-ordinates academic research into AIDS. Other bodies in Britain involved in AIDS research include

—The pharmaceutical industry

—The Department of Health and other health departments

—The Public Health Laboratory Service (PHLS)

—The National Institute for Biological Standards and Control (NIBSC)

—The Economic and Social Research Council (ESRC)

—The Central Office of Information (COI)

● **A Special Cabinet Committee** was set up in November 1986. It includes the Home Secretary, the Foreign Secretary, the Secretaries of State for Education, Defence, Social Services, Scotland, Wales and Northern Ireland.

● **An education campaign** began in January 1987, with a budget of £20 million. This included the use of television, newspapers, magazines, radio, posters and a leaflet drop to every home in order to reach as wide an audience as possible.

This campaign was aimed mainly at encouraging 'safer sex' with the use of condoms. The campaign literature does not state that condoms are free if obtained from a Family Planning Clinic. It also fails to mention the likely value of using a spermicide such as nonoxynol-9. Nonoxynol-9 kills herpes, chlamydia, gonorrhea and syphilis organisms, and also in laboratory experiments, the virus which causes AIDS. Though of unproven efficacy in actual use, it may be a valuable additional safety-net when used in conjunction with condoms. Other chemicals, such as benzalkonium chloride, may later prove to be better at killing viruses such as HIV, and once that is proven they should be strongly promoted.

Most importantly the campaign does not mention the failure rate of the condom. Thirteen to fifteen per cent of women using this as the sole means of contraception are pregnant within one year.

● **Surveillance** has been undertaken since 1982 with the PHLS Communicable Disease Surveillance Centre (CDSC), Colindale. AIDS cases are reported on an informal and voluntary basis to CDSC and to the Communicable Diseases (Scotland) Unit. Cases of HIV infection are also reported to CDSC on a voluntary basis.

In May 1985 all doctors in England were circulated with a DHSS booklet, *General Information for Doctors*, on AIDS. At this time there had been only 159 cases of AIDS reported in Britain.

● **All blood for transfusion has been tested** in Britain since October 1985. There is a new factory for the production of Factor 8, the blood component used for haemophiliacs.

• **HIV antibody testing**, using the ELISA test (see chapter 8), has been available since 1985 in Genito-urinary medicine/Sexually Transmitted Disease Clinics, and more recently in some hospital laboratories. This test is always preceded by counselling, and if the result is positive, follow-up counselling is provided. The result is not available to the patient's general practitioner or other medical people concerned in his or her care, unless the patient requests that it should be. HIV or AIDS is not a notifiable disease.

Britain and the Commonwealth

Britain is part of a family of nations, the Commonwealth, and has particular responsibilities to the member countries. There are forty-nine independent member countries within the Commonwealth, which contains almost a thousand million people, a quarter of the world's population.

Not only are we able to communicate through a common language, but to a great extent we also share the same pattern and principles of health care. Because of historical and personal links, Britain has particular opportunities to influence the course of the epidemic in many commonwealth nations, and therefore to help safeguard their future.

Each member country has a tremendous amount to offer the Commonwealth from its own experience and expertise. Commonwealth countries need to come together in open and frank discussion, each revealing their hopes and fears. They may issue suitable literature, exchange personal and educational programmes and give other support through the already well established Commonwealth Foundations.

Commonwealth countries recognize Queen Elizabeth as the symbol of the association and as Head of the Commonwealth. She is held in tremendous love and respect in this family of nations. A personal message from the Queen, perhaps on radio or television, would be an immensely powerful warning. Indeed it might be the greatest single factor in saving countless lives in many commonwealth countries.

International implications

Africa, North and South America, South-East Asia and Europe are all experiencing the AIDS epidemic. This could result in the weakening of these countries both in manpower and in social and financial cohesion.

In ten years' time the strong, stable countries will be those which have managed to contain the epidemic and preserve their population intact. The Soviet bloc countries, mainland China and the fundamentalist Muslim countries have both the politico-geographical barriers to prevent spread of infection and the totalitarian governments to take strong measures to contain infection if it does occur.

What of the Western countries? The education and public awareness campaign in the United States has succeeded in slowing down the rate of spread of HIV infection from the initial doubling time of five months to a doubling time of twelve months. This is of little comfort if numbers double from 3 million to 6 million in the space of one year, and to 12 million a year later. In fact the slowing effect could itself be a function of the time-distribution of the period during which the virus incubates and not a slowing of transmission at all. The United States may have done very little to alter the rate of transmission.

The Surgeon General of the United States, Everett Koop, has predicted that by 1991 there will be 270,000 cases of AIDS in the United States. If the ratio of people presenting with AIDS to those with HIV infection is still 1:50–100 at this time, this would represent between 13 and 26 million people infected with HIV by 1991 in the United States.

The figures in Europe can be seen from the table on page 81.

The AIDS future for Britain

Some have tried to soften the harsh impact of such figures. They have stated that, as in every other world epidemic in history, it would be truly surprising if the AIDS epidemic did not

- **Reach a ceiling by saturating a population;**
- **See the virus become less virulent as it is repeatedly passed on;**
- **Become checked by some treatment.**

If these three suppositions are examined in the light of history and what is known about the virus causing AIDS, it turns out that such comfort is illusory.

First, if a population is saturated by HIV it will be in the age range from eighteen to forty-nine, and there may be as many as 22 million people at risk in this age group in Britain. These include sexually

81

The Growth of an Epidemic

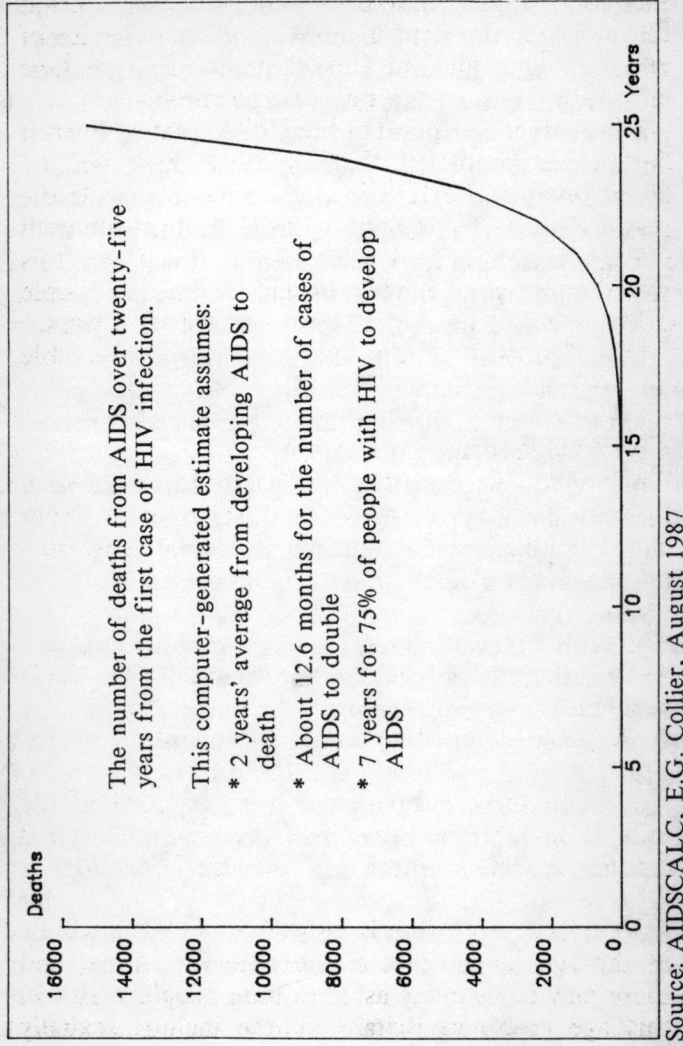

The number of deaths from AIDS over twenty-five years from the first case of HIV infection.

This computer-generated estimate assumes:

* 2 years' average from developing AIDS to death

* About 12.6 months for the number of cases of AIDS to double

* 7 years for 75% of people with HIV to develop AIDS

Source: AIDSCALC, E.G. Collier, August 1987

active homosexual males, married couples where
there are extramarital liaisons, men who visit prostitutes or who have occasional homosexual contacts,
intravenous drug addicts who share contaminated
needles and syringes, and wives, husbands, boy-
friends or girlfriends of any of those groups. Also at
risk are people who are divorced and, as it were,
become effectively single people again; and single
people searching for a permanent partner for life and
for whom 'serial monogamy' is a courting pattern.

This would mean that there are at least 34 million
people in Britain who have no apparent risk of
becoming infected with the virus. However, a satura-
tion of even one third of the people at risk in Britain
through their lifestyle would cause major damage to
society. Now remember this damage will affect
mainly those aged between eighteen and forty-nine.
This is going to be reflected in a depletion of the
numbers born in the next generation, as many who
would have been the parents of families will be lost.

Second, if we look at previous plagues in history
we see that the causative organism has not necessarily
achieved its maximum virulence in the early years of
the outbreak. In the most recent pandemic, the
1918-19 influenza which affected over a billion
people and killed 22 million in the space of twelve
weeks, a mild outbreak had occurred six months
before the main epidemic.

Other plagues lasted a long period of time, such as
the Plague of Justinian which lasted over a century
from AD 542 and killed 100 million. In three years
from 1346 the Black Death was thought to have
killed 37 million people in the East and 25 million in

the West. It is assumed that the Black Death was bubonic plague, and the pattern with bubonic plague is that it may be endemic in an area for many years after the initial severe outbreak, perhaps even for several hundred years with occasional epidemics of plague breaking out. By analogy with the above, it is possible that HIV has not yet achieved its maximum virulence. Similarly, there is no evidence to show that cholera, smallpox, tuberculosis or measles have become attenuated with time.

And third, there is at present no cure and no vaccine for AIDS. Although certain drugs such as AZT do have an effect on the virus by acting on the reverse transcriptase enzyme to prevent the virus replicating, this has unpleasant side effects. It is also expensive, costing between £10 and £15 for each day of treatment. And the person may need a blood transfusion every six to eight weeks. If the drug is stopped, the virus is then able to continue multiplying. AZT may therefore be said to prolong life, but it is not a cure. This drug may need to be given continuously for many months or years at an annual cost of between £5,400 and £7,000 for each patient.

So we need to look a major epidemic full in the face and find policies to cope with it, rather than look for false comfort.

What if the best happens, or the worst?
It is not yet known what course the AIDS epidemic in Britain will eventually take. But we have to prepare for the very real possibility that the pattern of HIV infection will change from Pattern One (predominantly homosexuals, intravenous drug

abusers and haemophiliacs) to Pattern Two (heterosexual spread), as has happened in Haiti and is beginning to happen in the United States.

The course of the epidemic in Britain will largely depend on whether a rapid change in lifestyles occurs and on the effectiveness of measures to prevent spread of the virus.

There are a number of different ways in which the population may be affected, which makes it dangerous to fix on facile 'definite figures'. It is more useful to look at the 'best situation' and the 'worst situation' with their implications.

● **The 'best situation'** will occur if the current education campaign is totally successful and lifestyles change so that chastity and faithful monogamous partnerships prevent further spread, and drug addicts no longer spread the virus by sharing infected needles and syringes. It assumes that prostitution ceases, and that the number of those infected with HIV in Britain remains at its present level estimated at up to 100,000.

● **The 'worst situation'** will come about if the virus continues to spread unchecked within the population. This will happen if lifestyles involving multiple sexual partners, extramarital relationships and certain homosexual practices do not change, if intravenous drug addicts continue to share infected needles and syringes, and prostitution still goes on. It may happen that the 'safer sex, use a condom' campaign either fails to be accepted, or if accepted only slows the rate of spread of HIV rather than stopping it.

If, in the worst possible situation, the numbers infected continue to double every nine months in Britain, then by 1991 there could be 3 million people infected, and by 1994, 12 million. At this point there would only be between 120,000 and 240,000 cases of AIDS in Britain. Most of the rest of the 12 million would be symptomless. But they would represent a time-bomb waiting to go off by the end of the century.

Britain is approximately four years behind the United States in the numbers infected with HIV. There are over 40,000 cases of AIDS in the United States according to the Center for Diseases Control in Atlanta. This represents the much larger figure of between 2 and 4 million people infected with the virus. However, in proportion to her population Britain is only two years behind the United States as by the end of 1989 one per cent of the population of Britain may have become infected with HIV.

The generation most at risk from the AIDS epidemic is the age group on which employment, creation of goods, wealth and services depend. It is the age group on which the defence of the country depends, the Armed Forces and the men and women who would mobilize in time of war. The production of the next generation of children depends on this generation, and an epidemic which reduces the numbers in this age range also weakens the country for the following generation.

If a large number of those aged from eighteen to forty-nine become infected with HIV and die of AIDS, then the economic base for the future is weakened. Also the ratio of working men and women to retired pensioners is reduced, at a time when the proportion of elderly people in the population would anyway be rising. And many elderly people will have no children to care for them.

The cost

It is thought that there may be as many as 100,000 people in Britain who are infected with HIV. As numbers are doubling every nine months at present, it is possible that within three or four years there could be 3 million people infected. It is not yet known what proportion of people infected with HIV will go on to develop AIDS and die, but experts are now talking in terms of from seventy-five to ninety per cent. If only seventy-five per cent of those infected develop AIDS, then estimates may be made of the costs to the country of an epidemic limited to 3 million infected with HIV with 2.25 million resulting deaths.

Costs include hospital treatment, which currently varies between £6,800 and £20,000 for each person. If twenty-five years of working life is lost for each person dying of AIDS, then the lost productive income comes to £612 thousand million.

As more than 160,000 children pass through the divorce courts each year into single-parent families, it is reasonable to suppose that many of these single parents might become infected as they search for a new partner. An arbitrary figure of 500,000 orphans has been taken as a possible number if 250,000 single parents are included in the number dying from AIDS.

In the same way, if 12 million become infected

with HIV, estimates may be made of costs to the country of 9 million deaths.

The total estimate runs out at £687 thousand million, as can be seen from the chart on page 89.

These are the costs if only seventy-five per cent develop AIDS of 3 million infected with HIV. If ninety per cent do, the figure gets correspondingly worse. The figure of £687 thousand million does not take into account the capital costs of providing new hospitals, hospices and so on, nor the cost of treatment with AZT. It does allow for the possible increased costs of law enforcement, long-term psychiatric care and other factors in a society where dementia and brain damage of varying degree affect a large number of young people.

But of course the best may happen. If the epidemic is halted and the numbers infected with HIV remain at, say, 100,000 and if we use the same assumption, the cost to Britain for hospital treatment will be £1,500 million and the cost of lost productive income £22,500 million, a total of £24,000 million. Because those infected early in the epidemic in Britain have in the main been homosexual males and at present few women are infected, any costs for caring for orphans would be small and may be discounted.

These would be the costs if the Zero-Option AIDS campaign is accepted and results in a widespread change of lifestyle.

Of course there is another way this 'best situation' could be achieved: by specific control measures of screening and separated living of those found to be antibody-positive. In that event the additional cost of housing at £40,000 each adds another £4,000 million, and the cost of screening the whole population twice yearly for fifteen years adds a further £1,500 million, making a total of £29,500 million.

The chart on page 89 shows how wide is the range of possible costs. And even scenario C is conservative. The worst possible figure is 9 million people with AIDS, which would cost £2,748 thousand million. This represents, at the current rate of spending on the National Health Service, the total NHS budget for 133 years!

What can be done?
There are three ways we can choose to go.

• **We can stay as we are.** We could choose to continue with an education campaign to encourage sexual restraint and use of condoms in at-risk situations, and to discourage the sharing of needles and syringes by drug addicts.

• **We can increase resources and attempt to limit the damage.** In this option we emphasize the safety of chaste lifestyles and faithfulness within marriage as giving no risk whatever of infection with HIV. ONE PERSON—ONE PARTNER FOR LIFE gives total safety and would be a 'Zero-Option AIDS' campaign. We also encourage widespread voluntary testing and institute a 'Zero-Option AIDS' campaign in schools, on television and at work.

For intravenous drug addicts 'new-for-old' needle—and syringe—exchange schemes could be instituted in a wide variety of venues, not just designated and experimental areas as at present.

What Will AIDS Cost?

(Figures in £million)

Scenario A: Voluntary change of lifestyle, no further infection

A: 24,000

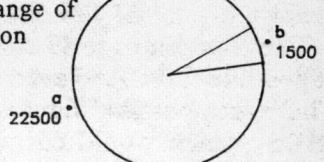

b
1500

a
22500

Scenario B: Specific control measures, no further infection

B: 29,500

d
4000

c
1500

b
1500

a
22500

Scenario C: AIDS continues unchecked; 75% HIV-positive contract AIDS

C: 687,000

e
30000

b
45000

a
612000

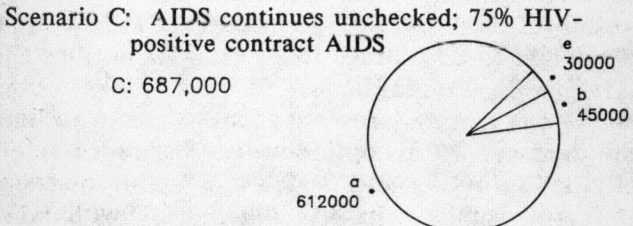

a - Lost productive income over 25 working years

b - Hospital treatment at £20,000 each

c - Screening of population twice-yearly for 15 years

d - Housing at £40,000 each

e - Care of orphans (estimated 50,000)

Health centres and pharmacies could be acceptable exchange-points. Schemes for drug addicts need to be flexible, with drug withdrawal as the eventual goal in addition to the availability of methadone programmes. Disciplined drug withdrawal programmes and methadone programmes also need a medical and social support component, in addition to advice on reducing the risk of spreading AIDS.

● **We can attempt to halt the epidemic by specific control measures.** These could include six-to-nine-monthly screening and separated living areas.

Specific measures to control the epidemic would reduce the rate of spread if successful. The first widespread screening would possibly identify 82,000 if 100,000 are already infected. Nine months later the remaining 18,000 would have doubled to 36,000, but 30,000 of these would be identified on this screening. The third screening would identify 10,000 leaving possibly 2,000 unidentified carriers of the virus because of the delay in developing antibodies to HIV until a few weeks after infection.

If, in addition to compulsory screening, seropositive people were required to live in a separate town or city, this would be a restriction on liberty unheard of in modern times. The nation would have to be seen to be facing a national crisis of death of the young generation on an unprecedented scale before such drastic measures would find acceptance.

Account would have to be taken of Britain's annual influx of 12 million visitors. Antibody-negative certificates could be required before entry, reinforced by a blood test, taking forty-five minutes and costing £2. The newest test to be developed needs only a few drops of blood and takes five minutes. This could be done on arrival at the port of entry.

At present in Britain we are at a relatively early stage in the epidemic in comparison with other countries. All three options justify serious consideration.

The threat

The potential danger to Britain and Europe of the AIDS epidemic may be as grave as a war situation. If we treat this plague with that degree of seriousness, then it is possible to face it with the firmness, strength and courage with which we would face a war.

Island Britain enjoys a unique geographical position in Europe. We may adopt preventive measures independently of Europe if we think it right. Our political independence is at least as important as our geographical separation. And we have greater flexibility than a political system with a constitution.

Measures to be taken are a political decision based on moral, economic, ethical and defence considerations. They must be acceptable within the framework of a democracy, and practical in that they must be possible to implement. They must be perceived as necessary and desirable for the whole of the population, not merely for a part of the population. It is wrong for measures to be taken solely for the benefit of those not infected, but it is equally wrong for measures to be taken, or not to be taken, solely for the benefit of those infected with the virus.

Ultimately the responsibility of government in a peacetime situation is to preserve the lives of its citizens. For those whose lives it is unable to preserve, its responsibility is to safeguard as good a quality of life as possible for the years which remain, and the best medical care. The fewer the people who are infected, the better the quality of care for sufferers will be. The medical care which can be given to 100,000 people is clearly greater than that which can be given to 3 million in the same length of time. So preventive medicine is even more important for AIDS than for medicine in general.

The 'worst' and 'best' situations and the various options which may be taken need to be evaluated as a matter of urgency. Global strategies designed in 1985, when it was thought that only ten per cent of those infected with the virus would develop AIDS and die, may no longer be appropriate in a situation with a possible ninety per cent mortality.

What follow are definite proposals for government action. They have been sent as an open letter to government and those in many areas of leadership. If implemented, they would at least tilt the epidemic into a less severe mode of operation.

Proposals to Government

We propose that the British government should:

1. **Declare AIDS to be a priority of the first rank in the country.**
2. **Review the basic strategy behind all efforts to combat the epidemic.**
3. **Lay emphasis in education campaigns on One Person, One Partner For Life,** which means chast-

ity, fidelity and protective friendship. This is valid worldwide and gives the only Zero-Risk AIDS.

4. Provide easy access to HIV testing for the general public and for doctors.

5. Remove as far as possible all financial disadvantages facing HIV-positive people who are still healthy, as at present this makes people resistant to being tested.

6. Reverse the current policy of negative counselling to dissuade people from having the test.

7. Encourage education on AIDS from an early age in school. Initially this can take the form of geographical and historical aspects of the epidemic, with indications that it is possible to choose a no-risk lifestyle.

8. Massively increase government funding for AIDS, to cover education on AIDS; expansion of medical services including hospitals, home care and hospices; and programmes aimed specifically at drug addicts and prostitutes.

9. Assist voluntary bodies with funding since these are expected to be in the forefront of caring for those suffering from AIDS-related conditions.

10. Generous government funding to an independent AIDS body with responsibility for Third World countries.

For further reading

(All these books and papers were published between 1985 and 1987 except where otherwise stated.)

AIDS: Meeting the Community Challenge, St Paul's Press

AIDS: Some Guidelines for Pastoral Care, Church House Publishing

AIDS and You: An Illustrated Guide, British Medical Association

AIDS Newsletter, Bureau of Hygiene and Tropical Diseases

AIDS Study Pack, Shaftesbury Project

Grosse Paul, *AIDS: Proposals for Action, the global epidemic and the crisis in Africa*

House of Commons Social Services Committee, *Problems Associated with Aids*, Memoranda, HMSO

McCloughry Roy, *AIDS: A Christian Response*, Shaftesbury Project

McKie Robin, *Panic: The Story of AIDS*, Thorsons National Working Party on Health Service Implications of HIV Infection, Report, HMSO

Office of Health Economics, *The AIDS Virus: Forecasting its Impact*, HMSO

Panos Dossier, Panos Institute

Rayner, Claire, *Safe Sex*, Sphere Books, London
Scottish Committee on HIV Infection and
Intravenous Drug Misuse, *HIV Infection in
Scotland*, Report, Scottish Home and Health
Department
Scottish Health Education Group, *Drugs and
Young People in Scotland*, published by the
authors
Slack Paul, *The Impact of the Plague in Tudor and
Stuart England*, Routledge and Kegan Paul
Ziegler Philip, *The Black Death*, Penguin, 1969
Zinsser Hans, *Rats, Lice and History*, Macmillan,
1934

More from Lion Publishing: